A Caregiver's Winding Road

Also by Jeannie Thomas:

Conscious Aging: Aging and End of Life Resources and Checklists

A Caregiver's Winding Road

An Insider's Guide to Courageous Caregiving

❦

Jeannie Thomas

Thomas Enterprises
530c Alameda Del Prado, #194
Novato, CA 94949

Thomas, Jeannie
A Caregiver's Winding Road: An Insider's Guide to Courageous Caregiving

ISBN 978-0-9839475-0-9

Jeannie Thomas is available for keynote speeches as well as half-day and full-day workshops. Contact us for rates and scheduling details.

www.CaregiversNook.com

Dedicated to my son
Chris Pessy
who by his loving kindness
enthusiasm for life
and delightful humor
brings me immeasurable joy

Contents

Acknowledgements

‿

MY DEEP GRATITUDE TO THE ELDERLY and the dying who touch my life. You teach me—not only about the end of life, but also the value of living well now, in this precious moment.

Disclaimer

ALTHOUGH THE INCIDENTS IN THESE stories are true, the names, locations and specifics of the situations have been changed. Additionally, some stories may be composites of several experiences.

The author of this book does not dispense medical advice nor prescribe the use of any technique as a form of treatment for medical problems.

This material is not intended to replace the advice of a qualified financial planner, attorney, tax adviser, investment professional or insurance agent. Before making any financial commitments, the appropriate professional should be contacted.

No part of this publication may be reproduced or transmitted in any form by any means, electronic or mechanical, including photocopy, recording or any information storage and retrieval system now known or to be invented, without permission and in writing from the publisher, except by a reviewer who wishes to quote brief passages in connection with a review written for inclusion in a magazine, newspaper or broadcast. Contact us at www.CaregiversNook.com.

PART 1

~

The Tough Questions

The Tough Questions

*I*NEVER INTENDED TO WORK WITH THE elderly and the dying. In the late 1980s, after leaving corporate management, I made a huge career leap and trained in massage therapy. I was happily self-employed and I loved everything I was doing. I made enough money to support my teenage son and myself and enjoyed the long-sought-after-luxury of making my own schedule. In 1995, this wonderful career was interrupted by an auto accident. During my recovery, my ability to work was limited for a number of years. I suffered from extreme pain in my neck and right shoulder that prevented me from performing my regular duties as a massage therapist.

During this time, my friend, Connie, approached me about taking care of her neighbor. Helen had bone cancer and required aid 24 hours a day. I was hired to stay with her during the night. It was a simple job in the beginning. Helen was a very petite woman who was a fall risk, so I basically stayed near her side and assisted her if she needed help. I also responded to her needs for pain medicine.

I stayed with this woman for several months and was by her side when she died. Her life touched me deeply and her story is included in the pages that follow.

After Helen passed away, I contacted an Agency about working with them. I had gained enough experience to pass their Health and Hygiene tests and applied for their CPR and First Aid classes.

As I grew in experience and reputation as a caregiver, I often found work through personal referrals. For years, this work sustained me financially and gave me purpose.

The stories and information that follow are an outgrowth of working with the elderly, the dying, their families and caregivers for over 15 years. As a caregiver for the elderly and the dying, I walked through many situations that surprised, shocked and scared me. In city after city in which I worked, there were huge numbers of elderly who needed help. Some lived fairly active lives. Most did not. Some had money. Some did not. Some had their memories and could care for themselves. Others could not. Many were alone much of the time.

With some clients, I visited them a few times a week. In other situations, I lived at their homes 24/7. I have cared for clients with pulmonary disease, blindness, cystic fibrosis, various types of cancer, dementia, Parkinson's, respiratory failure, multiple sclerosis, and Alzheimer's disease. I have worked in pre and post-op care. I have cared for amputees and paraplegics. I've changed diapers on a 280-pound man, washed feeding tubes, ran a comb through matted hair, used bathrooms that reeked of urine. One time a drunken daughter locked me out of her home: I was stranded outside with her invalid mother who was sitting in a wheelchair on a hot 98-degree day.

All my training was "on the job training." I've done things I never thought I'd be capable of doing. Just as many people today are suddenly thrown into the care of their aging parents or another family member, I walked into elder care unprepared for many of the experiences I was to encounter.

I did my best to begin my assignments knowledgeably. I found resources for "what to buy" and studied these and learned from them. When faced with caring for a person with a disease that I did not understand, I often spent many nights searching the Internet for answers to my questions. I went to therapy where I learned to "take good care of myself."

Nothing really prepared me for what I was to experience. Nothing prepared me for the decline of the body. Nothing prepared me for the sense of loss family members experience when a loved one is rapidly changing before their eyes.

I listened to the sadness of those suffering when spouses could no longer hold a glass in their hands, walk by themselves, or brush their own teeth. I sat with those who wept when their mother or father no longer recognized them. I held hands with spouses in so much pain they could not be in the room as their loved one died.

In my initial work with the elderly and the dying, my primary focus was on relieving pain and providing safety and comfort to those placed in my care. I often became very personally involved: a trait that is my gift as well as my nemesis. In my own defense, may I say that separating my heart and spirit from my work—especially work as deeply personal as caring for those in their last days—seems unconscionable to me.

As I became proficient in my duties, more knowledge-able in the various diseases afflicting those in my care and more comfortable taking charge in another's home, I began to participate in other aspects in these situations that had before eluded me. Once I became comfortable and skilled in working with the elderly I became more involved in communicating effectively with their loved ones. As my own mother became seriously ill, my learn-ing took on yet another deeper layer of growth. Now I was the one who needed advice, comfort and direction.

Sitting by the bedside of elderly patients in hospi-tals taught me that it is often customary these days for people to take doctor's orders as the final word in any given situation. Few of us question what the medical profession offer. In being with an aging and/or ill spouse or parent, often there are so many unwanted emotions that are being processed that we make decisions blindly. And—quite frankly—few people have the energy, time or outside support to seek alternative answers to their concerns.

It was becoming more and more apparent to me, that—like raising a child—there are no guidebooks to help us navigate the winding road of aging and dying.

Born between the years 1946 and 1964, I am what the statisticians call a baby boomer. It is projected that in the not-so-distant future, when the baby boomers come into their Golden Years, there will be 72 million of us. According to the U.S. Census Bureau, there are now about 100,000 centenarians in the United States. That population is rapidly growing. The Bureau projects by 2050 there will be 1.1 million centenarians in America alone. Meanwhile, researchers at an East Coast University predict there will be even more, estimating some 3 million baby boomers will live to be 100 or older.

Aside from extreme medical advances, these statistics beg the question: What does the future hold for the aging and the dying baby boomers? If only one percent of the projected 72 million of us are using walkers to ambulate, this translates to 720,000 people with walkers. A staggering figure!

Already, we are seeing the signs of a changing population. Nursing and Retirement Homes are being filled as quickly as they are being built. Items that used to be relegated to a medical pharmacy are available at the local drugstore: adult diapers and walking canes are as common as aspirin. You can purchase a vehicle that you drive around your living room through a National Television advertisement.

And who will care for the aging and the dying? In order to financially survive as a caregiver, one needs to be either totally financially independent or share housing with another. In my own case, as a single woman, I downsized my life to the minimum requirements, not something most people are willing to do.

As I watched families flounder through the experience of their parents' aging and dying, I often witnessed their lives taken to the brink of emotional and financial ruin. Often, the first step is to try and care for the loved one without moving them from their surroundings. Missed work, hours in traffic and the stress of trying to run two homes take a tremendous toll on daily life. Marriages suffer and family life becomes non-existent.

The next step might be to hire a caregiver. Thus begins the interview process. Unless you have the good fortune to know someone you trust, this can be a daunting experience. No matter the references, you really don't know how the caregiver will function in your particular situation. There are so many variables: the temperament of your loved ones, the nature of their illness, the stage of their illness and the rapport with other family members, to name but a few. And there are other questions: Can the caregiver cook? Maintain cleanliness? Be trusted when she/he is not under your watchful eye?

Hiring a caregiver through an Agency requires due diligence. It's important to know how to use an Agency effectively. I have worked for several and all companies are not equal. In some instances, if staff is short, a client might be assigned the first available caregiver. This could mean that the caregiver actually has little experience in the skills you are seeking. I received many calls from Agencies asking if I "would be willing to learn" various important functions, i.e., "… how to clean a catheter … how to move a paraplegic … how to deal with a late stage Alzheimer's client." It's important to ask the right questions when researching Agencies so that you are not at their mercy.

I have personally been told to leave a compromising situation once the client's money ran out. In some circumstances, typically hospice, if a person's "vitals" change, care may no longer be covered by Insurance. I felt sickened one time when I was told to leave a woman who was bed bound. She had dementia and had no idea that she could not walk. She would grab the side rails of the hospital bed and force herself over them, landing harshly on the floor, her oxygen tube yanked from her face, now tangled around her hands and arms. She was left to the mercy of the Retirement Home's staff to check on her from time to time.

Granted, these are not the "norm", or so one would hope. And I am not here to bash any caregiver, agency, family member, medical practitioner or paid professional. Their work is thankless and difficult. In many cities, there is a shortage of help, so the ones providing care are often over-worked and stressed beyond their limits. Burnout is common. A paid caregiver does not make much money. On the other hand, only the elite wealthy can afford the wages of hiring a caregiver who "lives in" 24/7.

Other options for care involve families moving in together. In other situations, homes are sold to support their loved one being moved into a Retirement Home.

If the elder person becomes very ill, the next step may be a Nursing Home. Becoming more and more popular is the concept of a facility that has it all: private apartments or cottages, retirement apartments, assisted living arrangements, and, additionally, nursing facilities.

There are no easy answers to the complexities involved as one ages. Facing death is personal and internal and ominous and still remains a subject many do not want to discuss. There are no easy answers for the myriad of situations facing the elderly, the dying and their caregivers.

I hold in my heart a great amount of respect for those who walk gracefully through their own difficult process of aging and dying.

I am humbled by the adult children, grandchildren, caregivers, agencies, paid professionals, conservators, doctors, nurses, hospice volunteers and families whose lives are ultimately and significantly affected by the aging and the dying.

On a deeply personal level, my experiences have forced me to look at my own aging and dying in a manner that never before occurred to me.

These questions went far beyond the "life support issues" that one considers when completing those little pink forms that get magnetized to our refrigerators for paramedics in case of an emergency. I questioned if I would I opt to use oxygen 24 hours a day. If I needed kidney dialysis three times a week, how would this affect my quality of life? If my blood circulation weakened, would I want toes, feet or even limbs amputated? If my bladder had cancer, would I opt to have it removed and urinate through a tube in my stomach?

What about our medical community's responsibility? Most of the elderly who were in my care were on a minimum of 20 prescriptions. Many of these drugs have serious side affects. Many of them clash internally in the bodies of those they are supposed to help. How much is modern medicine merely keeping our bodies functioning at a very minimal level? How often is the patient's "quality of life" considered? And how does one define quality of life? What does that actually mean to each person?

What does quality of life mean to me? Who determines its meaning?

Here, again, I do not intend to bash the medical community. We are blessed with brilliant medical practitioners and a myriad of marvelous pharmaceuticals. Co-operating with them wisely is a choice that we have.

The stories that follow are the culmination of some of my deepest experiences caring for the elderly and the dying. With these stories I honor those whose lives I shared in their final days. I honor those who stand by their loved ones, caring for them through the ever-changing process of aging and dying. As you read their stories, I hope you will glean some insights into the daily lives of those you know and love that may be aging or in the process of dying.

If you are now a caregiver, perhaps you will uncover in Part 3 a much-needed way of coping that will assist you through your personal process.

In my second book, "Conscious Aging," I offer a buffet of resources: no one among us needs to travel this road alone and there are many tools and organizations to help us along the way.

My two manuscripts are intended for the caregiver, the aging and their family members. Hopefully, all will benefit.

As you peek through the windows of my own experiences, perhaps you, too, will be inspired to share your situations, your solutions and your beliefs. No one publication can provide all the questions or answers. I hope that this book and the subsequent blog will be the beginning of an ongoing dialog surrounding the realities and the mysteries of aging and dying.

Please access our blog to air your concerns and to support others. If you have questions about the situation in which you are involved, reach out so that others may offer their experience. If you have mixed emotions about what you are experiencing, may you find permission for self-expression and personal acceptance. If you have discovered a new way of coping—or even a new product that's helped in your situation—please "pass it on" and share it with us.

I hope that knowing you are not alone will open the door to an honest and profound sharing of your experiences so that together we can find strength, comfort, and hope.

Jeannie Thomas
September 2011

~

Share your story, your concerns and your solutions:
www.CaregiversNook.com

Hidden in America

*T*HEY ARE EVERYWHERE. YET NO ONE SEES them...

They may be your neighbors.
Or your co-worker's Mother.

They live in million dollar estates and in one-room apartments.
They are among the wealthiest and the poorest.

Some speak. Some do not.

Some will hear you. Others are deaf.

They are lonely. And alone.
Many are confused and frightened.

They feel sad, angry, blessed, sorrowful, strong, helpless, happy, alone, delighted, depleted, frightened, forgotten, loved, scorned, respected, weak or wonderful.

Some have forgotten who they are.

They are America's elderly.
Many are very ill. Many are dying.
They are everywhere. Yet no one sees them ...

Their caregivers could be close friends or family members.
They could be strangers hired by referral or through
  Agencies.
These caregivers give without hope for validation.
They often toil without taking time for meals.
They have many sleepless nights.
They feel sad, angry, blessed, sorrowful, strong, helpless,
  happy, alone, delighted, depleted, frightened, forgot-
  ten, loved, scorned, respected, weak or wonderful.

They are everywhere. Yet no one sees them ...

PART 2
Personal Stories

~

The Elderly
and
the Dying
I Have Loved

Bone Cancer

*H*ELEN HAS BEEN BED-BOUND FOR ABOUT three months now. She's a widow with two children, both of whom live several States away from her. Her son, Michael, is a building contractor and Spring is a busy time of year for his business. Daughter Susan teaches Sixth Grade at an Illinois Middle School. Besides demanding jobs, both son and daughter have children of their own, and, soccer practice, dance lessons and homework make for busy lives. Michael and Susan have offered Helen a refuge in their homes for her final days. She does not want to go to them and has refused both their offers. They cannot come to her.

Financially, it's a "plus" that Helen's home is completely paid for. She lives in a well-kept older middle class neighborhood in a three-bedroom home where Michael and Susan were raised.

There are few signs that she is dying and her home neither feels nor smells like an over-used hospital room. Although the furnishings are a vintage 20 years, the home still flaunts a neat and clean appearance: one that is neither too old nor very new. A curved archway introduces the dining room. Bull-nose corners give the dwelling a soft easy feeling. The newer Berber carpet adds a more contemporary touch. So does the window in the living room that faces the backyard. The original standard box-framed windows were gutted several years ago when Helen's spouse, Jim, was still alive. The replacement is one large entire glass wall that lets in the sight of a well-manicured lawn, bright bushes of glorious roses and a side yard border of tall cypress trees stretching heavenward. Local hummingbirds poke at the colored liquid that Helen dutifully provides for them.

The only equipment in her home that appears medical is her walker. It's been around for a few years. Other than this, Helen's home is bereft of a hospital bed, a bed side table, stool softeners, "Depends", handy-wipes, grab bars: all the typical surroundings of one who is home alone and dying.

Helen spends most of her days slumbering in a chair in the living room. She grows weaker each day yet she is too proud to have a wheelchair brought into the home. I assist her when she needs to move from one place to another. She grabs anything she believes will hold weight: her mahogany desk, the arm of a chair, a brass door handle. This is not a safe way to maneuver. Never having been a large person, her five foot four inch frame now only carries 80 pounds, so it is easy for me to assist her to the toilet and to a chair at her sturdy oak kitchen table.

I've been hired for the night shift and have a simpler job than most of the other caregivers. Even though it is past her mealtime when I arrive, if Helen wants something to eat, I prepare food for her. I encourage her to drink water.

She is a fall risk, so I assist her to the bathroom. Cleaning herself afterwards is impossible. That's also my job. She's already in her warm checkered nightgown when I arrive, so there is no need to bathe or shower her unless she soils herself. Helen is non-complaining about her situation.

I know, she knows, everybody knows that her condition is terminal.

This is not only my first experience with Hospice; it is my first experience caring for the elderly. I, a stranger to Helen, am the person with whom she spends her final days. I may actually be the person by her side when she dies.

It is an auspicious place to be: helping a stranger through a terminal illness during her final days on earth. I ask myself what I can actually **do** to provide care and comfort for Helen that might be meaningful. I am keenly aware that whatever I do I must stay very **present.**

Working with one who is this close to death, I realize that we are not going to be talking about any future plans and perhaps not even past experiences. The dying need

> I gamble that the best game plan is none.

to let go of everything: their loved ones, their memories, their surroundings, and all their possessions. Finally, they need to drop their own flesh and blood, their container that's been with them since birth. A daunting challenge.

I quickly realize that my previous training in massage therapy may be of little value in my new situation. However, years of learning to touch others with care and compassion has taught me a few valuable lessons. I gamble that the best game plan is none. I keep my attention focused on what's in front of me. I tell myself: "Stay in the moment. Respond in the moment. Let go of my own ideas of what should or should not be done. Trust my intuition."

In an attitude of intending to comfort, I re-arrange the living room, placing Helen's favorite chair in a direction that affords her views of the beautiful California sunlight as it filters through the sheer curtains and onto the two porcelain waltzing figurines which adorn her sparse coffee table.

I bring several vases to her home. Each day I choose a fresh rosebud from her garden and position it where she can enjoy the petals as they gently open to greet her. On very warm days, one of the special hybrids emits a magnificent scent. The delight this brings Helen is palpable and brings a smile to my face.

The sense of smell is very acute in the dying and even though her appetite is meager, I bake goodies that send the sweet aroma of vanilla or cocoa wafting through the air. Simple pleasures.

As Helen's illness progresses, the doctors have ordered morphine for her pain.

Because I am paid directly by the family, with their permission I can administer medication. The morphine can be given every four hours as needed for pain. For the first couple of days, Helen's pain is alleviated through two doses of morphine: one in the morning and one in the evening. She closes her eyes, opens her mouth and swallows the distasteful liquid. Twice a day is a sufficient dosage to assuage her pain.

However, as the days wear on, her pain increases. So does the morphine.

Helen begins a barely audible mantra praying, "God, please take me."

In a world where *"doing"* is idolized, I am faced with the reality that right now, in these last moments with Helen, there really is nothing to do. This is a time of simply *"being"* with her. My offerings to and for her are those of my spirit. I go deep within myself to access a willingness to be fully present for her. I stand by her side in a manner of holding her in comfort. I offer my care for her ... a deep longing that she may find peace and that she may transition gracefully.

I offer her all of my love as if I have known her for a lifetime. She allows me the gift of being by her side during this, the most auspicious time of her life. In doing so, she honors me.

The last week of Helen's life, her suffering is too much for most of the caregivers.

New replacements arrive each day. One such replacement phones me in the middle of the day, begging me to come to her aid.

When I arrive, Helen, writhing in pain, is offering her mantra, "God, take me. Take me. God, please take me."

Today, Helen's pallor seems stark and bleached. Her skin seems stretched tight across her jaw. Her breathing is intensely labored. Her hair is matted and wet with sweat. Her unfocused eyes are dark as blackberries.

"She's dying," I whisper to the other caregiver. "Don't be afraid. Just be with her. We need to just be with her and hold her. There is nothing we have to do. Just **be** with her.

We need to let her know by our touch that we love her ... and we are here for her ... no matter what."

I whisper in Helen's ear. "It's okay. Just let go. You are safe. Do not be afraid."

As I speak to her and as we gently hold her, Helen's body begins to relax. The tension in her muscles begins to soften.

We stand on either side of her bed and wrap our arms around her. We hold her.

I stroke her forehead and her face like I would a small child's. I whisper to her, "It is okay. You are safe. Do not be afraid." This becomes *my* mantra.

At that moment, the most unlikely sound is heard. The phone by Helen's bedside is ringing. The only time the phone rings at this house is when Michael or Susan call their mother. In disbelief, I stare at the other caregiver, as if to ask, "*What in the world do we do now?*"

I decide to answer the call.

It is Helen's daughter, Susan, from Chicago on the other end of the line.

Unbelievable.

Since that afternoon, I've often wondered: do you think it's possible that some cosmic force binds us to those we love, sending out light waves of information as one passes from this life ... sending shining beams of love's rays from one heart to another ... sending signals across the miles that say, "I'm going now. I'm leaving. I just need to say 'Good Bye' to you."

"Susan." I speak softly. "Your mother is dying."

There is a profound silence as Susan tries to absorb what I am saying. Of course she and everyone knows that her mother is in the final stage of her life. I realize that she knows I am not telling her anything that she doesn't already know. She doesn't quite know what to make of my words to her. It's confusing.

"No," I say. "I mean, *She's Dying. Right Now. She Is Leaving Us This Very Moment.*"

Susan has the heart and presence of mind to ask that the phone be placed next to her mother's ear.

Helen, still begging to be taken by God, still gasping for air, finally begins to let go as the sound of her only daughter, Susan, whispers in her ear, "We love you so much, Mom. We love you so very much."

Helen's entire body, oh so slowly, deeply, softly relaxes as she lets go. One last sweet breath of life and she is gone.

Bent-Over Betty

ONE OF THE MOST ENDEARING WOMEN I've had the pleasure to meet thus far as a caregiver is Betty Burnley. Betty is 95. She wears nursing shoes and pants too long for her crippled legs. She has never worn glasses. Still, her aged sparkling liquid blue eyes have the eyesight of a hungry eagle. When she sees me, she dons a wide generous smile and I feel as if the sun has dawned for me alone.

One day while walking home from the grocery store, Betty takes a serious fall on the asphalt. She requires immediate medical attention and is sped away by ambulance to the nearest hospital. She has no known family, no friends. The Courts give her care and her money to a State appointed conservator. The conservator sends me to her home.

Betty has a hump on her back so pronounced, that, while standing, she looks like she is bent in half. To see me eye to eye, she has to arch her neck, bend her head completely backwards and stretch her eyes upwards toward her forehead. Betty is naturally so bent-over that when she climbs the flight of stairs to her second level apartment, her hands actually touch the cold step in front of her. She climbs deliberately and with caution reaching the small 1 room apartment she's inhabited for 35 years. Strolling into her abode, I see a rickety twin bed. A tired sunken sofa. A 15 inch black and white TV. A solitary washed-out brown chair. A tiny confining kitchen. A cramped bathroom.

Did you ever fall in love with someone because of her laughing eyes? You would adore Betty.

Betty eats the same meals every day, making it an easy task to memorize her weekly shopping list:

    1 can of pineapple juice
    1 box of oatmeal
    1 quart of milk
    1 small bunch of carrots
    1 head of celery
    1 head of cabbage
    1 loaf of bread
    1 package of cheese slices

This is Betty's breakfast every day:

    Oatmeal with milk
    1 glass of pineapple juice

This is Betty's lunch every day:

    Cheese on bread

This is Betty's dinner every day:

    Boiled carrots, celery and cabbage

Betty never learns to drive a car. She never marries. She has no social circle. To earn a living, Betty cared for the children of working parents. She's saved almost $100,000 from her life's work changing diapers and wiping soiled mouths.

I am paid to take Betty to lunch today. She is so excited that she greets me dressed in a bright orange polyester suit that I'm sure she hasn't worn in 30 years. I feel royally honored. She sports a wide perennial smile on her little worn wrinkled face. Did you ever fall in love with someone because of her laughing eyes? You would adore Betty.

Because Betty has a bank account that will sustain her for the rest of her lifetime, the conservator decides to move her into a Retirement Home. At Golden Gardens, Betty will have a new room and three full meals a day. She is enticed by the prospect of a wonderful *new* menu every day. Apples, eggs, biscuits, ham, sweets! Oh, those yummy chocolate cakes and creamy tapioca puddings!

Preparing to move Betty from her apartment, the conservator instructs me to pack her belongings. As I do, I discover a purse filled with several thousand dollars of cash. I pack the purse in a box with other personal items. The conservator has trusted men on staff who regularly move her clients. They load the boxes into a van and unpack Betty's belongings at her new home. When Betty and I arrive at her new apartment, the purse is there. The money is not.

It only takes a single day to pack, move, unpack and set up Betty in her new home. 95 years old, and, after 35 years in one small room, Betty is more terrified than elated in her new surroundings. I'm exhausted. My workday is done, but I can't leave frightened Betty alone. I brush her grey locks. I gently massage her tired tiny bony feet. I tuck her in bed like I would a small child. She slips into sleep. She sleeps well.

I sleep curled up on Betty's small stiff sofa with a bath towel over me to keep me warm. It's been a good day.

↩

The conservator has directed me to visit Betty every day for a week. Learning that she always eats alone while others join their friends, I opt to share meals with her. I arrive, scan the huge dining room, and see her bent-over body sitting all alone at a large table set for six. Her aloneness is palpable. She›s all dressed up in her orange polyester suit and does not quite fit into the uppity elder caste inhabiting Golden Gardens. Her eyes light up when she sees me as she "puts her glow on." She looks beautiful.

One week after our initial meal together at the Retirement Facility, the conservator instructs me not to visit Betty anymore, fearing she will get too attached to me. There are others who need immediate care. Having formed a close relationship with her, and, caring deeply for her, I feel ripped off. How can I become so intimately involved in this person's life and walk away without feeling I am betraying her? I can›t imagine how Betty feels.

This new arrangement seems so unnatural to me. But I am not in the conservator's shoes and I am inexperienced in making choices in this arena.

A few days pass. Late one night the phone rings. It's the conservator. Without emotion, she chops out the news that Betty is in Intensive Care. She›s had a heart attack and is not expected to live. No matter the midnight hour,

I must see her. I race to her hospital room and arrive as quickly as I can. Being her only guest and feeling guilty about withdrawing from her life, I kneel by her bedside and begin to weep.

In a shaky weepy voice, I attempt to apologize. "I am so incredibly sorry I have not seen you. This was not my idea. But I could have come. I am so very very sorry. I could have come."

With only minutes of life remaining in her frail frame, her raspy little voice begins to choke from her now-broken body. Betty, gasping as she labors to speak, rolls her head towards me, whispering: "I know you love me…" Those lovely liquid blue eyes of hers meet my tear-filled ones. She gently squeezes my hand, closes her eyes and breathes her last precious breath.

Cirrhosis of the Liver

S TEPPING INTO THIS EXQUISITE ESTATE IN
the hills of Malibu, I feel as if I have stepped into
an ancient walled Italian city. Each room exudes elegant beauty and old country charm. The ornate entry
is domed with a stunning rotunda that Michelangelo
himself would have been proud to claim as his creation.
Thick walls are washed in brushed gold. Ornate paintings,
heavy tapestries and winged angels bless the eyes at every
turn. A spiral granite staircase sweeps me upstairs to a
rich haven where I will spend my nights.

A large room downstairs is my workspace during the
day. Here lays bed-bound Madeline.

Amidst the thick folds of an expensive quilted comforter, I spot the catheter tube that dangles to the bag
below. The unsightly bag is always in plain view so that I
can tell if it needs to be emptied. A testament to her failing body, it swells with dark urine. I unclip the bag and
walk to the bathroom and as I empty its contents I sing
a little song to myself. "Que sera sera … whatever will
be, will be …" Singing gets me through the task without

feeling sick to my stomach. Dealing with foul urine and smelly human feces is a big part of my job. I've never gotten use to this.

Madeline no longer experiences bowel movements since she's been given a liquid diet for almost an entire month.

An oxygen tube runs from her nostrils to the huge tank in the living room.

Shuuusssh. Clunk. Shuuussh. Clunk. Shuuusssh. Clunk.

There is no respite from the mechanical sound of the metal box that keeps Madeline alive. Even though it is two rooms away, the constant sound of the oxygen machine never becomes white noise. No lit matches, please.

Madeleine isn't expected to live another week.

This slight bed-bound woman is only in her mid-fifties. She looks 70. Her papery yellow skin is blotched with bruises where needles have attempted to administer food or pain relievers into her stick-like limbs. She cannot take the slightest touch without her skin quickly coloring into purple and black wrinkled pools. Her eyes are deep dark sumps of fresh congealed anger. Her scalp is sticky with shocks of grey clumps of prickly hair.

She has a lovely gentle daughter, Carley, and a wonderful affectionate son, Steven. Her husband, Jerome, has the patience of Job and dotes on her as if she is God's gift to mankind.

Shuuusssh. Clunk. Shuuussh. Clunk. Shuuusssh. Clunk.

Madeline has cirrhosis of the liver. She didn't catch cirrhosis. She doesn't have a genetic propensity that brought about her disease. In Madeline's case, the poisoning of her liver is the direct result of extreme hatred towards herself that manifested itself as alcoholism. She voted for it.

The liver is an amazing organ and is absolutely necessary for one's survival. It controls infections. It processes hormones and nutrients. It's a great cleaning agent, removing toxins and bacteria from the blood. It's a large organ, and, when healthy, possesses amazing regenerative properties. It is my understanding, that there are circumstances when you can ruin part of your liver, replace your destructive habits with healthy ones, and the remains of your liver will happily regenerate: "Voila!" You've got a new liver.

With end stage cirrhosis, all bets are off. Damaged cells can't be replaced. In Madeline's case, cirrhosis sends her in a downward spiral taking her psyche and her body to the depths of hell.

The Chinese believe that organs are connected to certain emotions in the body. They believe that the liver governs anger. I don't know if there is any truth to this theory, but I will say that I have never met anyone angrier than an alcoholic with cirrhosis. Madeline, lying in bed on death's door, a catheter at one end of her body, tubes down the other end, is the angriest woman I've ever met. Her lovely daughter and wonderful son come into her room with clenched jaws and stiff backs. They dread visiting her. Outside her room, they whisper between themselves. Like the terrorized victims that they are, they keep hoping and wishing for a few crumbs of love from their dying Mother.

This will never happen.

Madeline yells orders at her husband constantly. He crawls in and out of her room, the passive look of "the beaten" smeared across his dull white face. She hollers. He appears. She yells. He runs quickly to do her bidding. I have no doubt they've been dancing this dance for the full 30 years of their marriage. I am embarrassed for him. Yet he seems comfortable in some strange robotic way.

Before meeting Madeline, I believed that most people soften as they approach the final moments of their lives. I muse that some strange and wonderful forgiveness washes through them: for others and for themselves. I can almost hear their inner Louis Armstrong singing, "It really was a wonderful life. Sure, I had my ups and downs. But all in all, it was a beautifully wonderful life."

But Madeline never softens. No matter the tender gentleness from her daughter, the loving kindness from her son, the constant attention from her husband. No matter the music or the sunshine. No matter that she is shortly leaving this earth and will never see any of them again.

It's a rare situation in my experience when a dying person wants nothing.

There seems to be nothing I can do to offer comfort to Madeline. She flinches from even the smallest offering of human contact. I need to forgo all offerings of solace. This weighs heavily on me and feels contrary to the natural human stirrings within my heart.

It's a rare situation in my experience when a dying person wants nothing: no soft touch, no massage of the hands or feet, no stroking of the face, no words of comfort, not even the presence of family. What to do? I become quiet inside and listen for an answer to my question. The message comes, "Talk to her spirit in silence. Pray for her spirit in the quiet. Speak to her spirit with words of hope and gentleness and kindness."

That is exactly what I do.

In the inner sanctum of my heart, I speak to her, "Madeline, you are safe. You are protected and all is well. Your life on this earth is almost over. But a new life awaits you that will feel light and sweet and serene. Your loved ones are here offering their comfort and their care. You are well loved. You may not feel this now. But soon you will know this. You are deeply cared for. Many angels are here to help you transition to your new life. Surrender to their love. Surrender. It is time to let go now."

I have been brought into Madeline's life in the last few days she will spend on earth. Sitting by her bedside day and night for these three days, I beg heaven that her persona will soften. But she is bitter to the end. She never has a kind word for her husband or her children. She never seems happy when her son, her daughter or her husband walk into her room. It appears that she has never really loved anyone during her entire lifetime.

In some instances, as one approaches their last hours, a phenomena occurs known as "the death rattle." It is a peculiar sound that emanates from deep within the throat cavity as excess secretions accumulate. This usually begins within hours of a person's death and may even occur after a person dies. The gurgling sounds dry and wet at the same time. It has the noise of a broken rattle: dry bones hitting against each other in a ghostly wet wind.

Day three with Madeline. The death rattle begins. I have never heard it before.

It frightens me.

Madeline's death rattle lasts almost 24 hours. Her anger rages through her death rattle and hour after hour a hideous mean gurgle wells up from her failing flesh.

This is one of my longest days. Ever.

Shuuusssh. Clunk. Shuuussh. Clunk. Shuuusssh. Clunk.

Madeline's husband, Jerome, is in the garage when Madeline takes her last breath. It seems odd that he is not nearby. But perhaps not. Madeline dies as she had lived. Alone. Angry.

No one sheds a tear for her.

After she passes, I keep thinking, "Your life, Madeline? What was the point?"

Shuuusssh. Clunk. Shuuussh. Clunk. Shuuusssh. Clunk.

I stay with Madeline for a few minutes after she passes. I find Jerome and tell him that Madeline has died. He seems relieved.

"For God's sake, will someone please unplug that oxygen machine?" is all he says.

I unplug the machine, offer my condolences, leave quietly, walk through the front door, get into my car and begin the journey to my next assignment.

Rich Single Woman

$\mathcal{R}$ICH SINGLE WOMEN CAN BE FOUND LIV-
ing alone in beautiful upscale estates along the
Pacific Coast in California. I meet one such landowner
in a quiet seaside neighborhood in Cambria. Her ocean
view home has several sprawling patios each and every
one filled with potted geraniums in bright burgundy,
delicate pinks and shimmering whites. Her back yard
is a deep decadent declining hillside where tall pines
reach their arms to an adoring blue sky. Dancing metal
art and clear gazing balls dot the area near the largest of
the patios that is built on stilts over the backside of the
home. Fragrant sage borders the sides of the home while
wild orange lilies burst into flames to greet visitors. Deer
come at dusk to feed. If there is such a thing as paradise
on earth, this could be it.

The inside of the home is furnished tastefully, not lavish,
yet bears the mark of the rich. Black granite counter tops
in the kitchen. The current Wolff stove and oven. Thick
rich carpets the color of the sky splashed through the
living room. Here, also, are plush deep sofas from which

one can view the sea. The master bathroom sports a huge blue tiled shower built for six, a water closet complete with a red telephone and a cupid fountain set between two large sinks. The bathroom, by itself, is large enough and elegant enough to rent out as a vacation resort.

After my brief tour of the client's home, I am led to her room on the second floor. It's unusual to have someone who is ill or dying on a level other than the first floor, however, this situation is different: an elevator in the home rules out stairs being an issue. Her room has a spartan look—one often found in situations where someone has been bed-bound for a long time. No carpet here in order to accommodate first a walker, then a wheelchair.

The beautiful laced comforter and satin bedding have long since been replaced with a plastic lined mattress protector and easy-care linens. A table near the bedside is equipped with stool softeners, suppositories, diapers, Desitin, baby wipes, plastic gloves, hand cream, Vaseline, spare plastic bags, prescription medicines, a glass of water and a can of Ensure. Family pictures are now placed on every available dresser or table space even though this woman no longer recognizes any of the faces that smile at her.

The woman I am about to meet had been a famous performer in "the day." I was not to be told her last name. No matter. Illness levels the playing field. Rich or poor. Humble or proud. Intelligent or weak-minded. All the lines that divide us disappear during a terminal illness. The present moment is all that matters. The present moment reigns. The present moment becomes *"All There Is."*

Even so, I am sure that my client is now unrecognizable from the days of her famous youth. She had been beautiful, accomplished, well known and loved. But that was in "the day."

When I enter the room to meet her, she is seated in a large over-stuffed leather reclining chair. Even from the back I can tell that several blankets are wrapped around her legs, not uncommon for the elderly whose circulation is often weak. As the feet are the furthest distance from the heart, they typically receive the least amount of oxygen and remain a constant icy cold temperature. I walk around the chair to greet her. I have seen many elderly people in varying states of demise. Yet nothing could have prepared me for the sight of this particular human being.

This woman's face is thin and drawn with bleak hollows for eyes. Her skin, once creamy and beautiful before a camera, is blotchy and black-marked with green pus-

I nickname her "Marlena" after the great Dietrich of that name.

filled sores oozing from her sunken cheeks. She has absolutely refused oral hygiene for years. She has a few dark teeth left in her withered mouth. If a tooth becomes sore or infected, a dentist is called to the home. He'll bring something to sedate her and proceed to pull the troubling tooth.

She has long wild grey-black hair that springs out in all directions. It is the perfect frame for her crusty face.

She has long thin fingers with thick grey nails that curl because she will not let anyone near her to trim them. Liver spots cover her hands and arms and speckle her 80-year old face. I would have figured her to be over 100 years old.

Her voice has a long drawn out affected quality to it that I ascribe to "Old Hollywood." I nickname her "Marlena" after the great Dietrich of that name.

In this elegant affluent home, Marlena slouches in an old tattered nightgown. Soft food is placed near her side and she scoops it up with her spindly fingers and stuffs it inside her mouth. Meals are served in large bowls or plates with raised edges so that she can thus feed herself without loosing too much food on the floor in the process.

Although she cannot see, Marlena can hear. The flat-screen television babbles on all day. "Fox News." "News" and more "News." I find this a common theme with the elderly, this craving the "News" all day and into the night. Does listening to it make them feel in touch with the world? Do they enjoy the drama of the reporters as they spew deeply tragic and emotionally packed stories? Does it somehow give them a false sense of belonging to the world? Or, perhaps, this is merely a long-standing habit.

No matter.

This once-famous, once-intelligent, once-talented woman has no control of her urine or her bowels and wets and defecates just like a baby in a huge big diaper. This elegant room reeks of urine and feces.

Marlena does not like me and she does not want me in her home. When I attempt to change her, she raises her long legs and feet, and, with surprisingly powerful force, kicks me dead-on in the stomach while cursing me with her vile angry mouth. Right from the start, I make it very clear to her that in no way will I tolerate such behavior.

I do not mince any words with her: "You can not speak to me this way. You might not like me. You might not like what I do. But I will not tolerate any mean behavior from you. You cannot swear at me. You cannot kick me. And no matter what you think of me, I am going to give you the best care that I can. I will treat you well. I expect you to treat me well. I am here to help you in any way that I can."

This surprises her. I suspect that no one has spoken to her in that way for a long time. We come to an agreement. Nothing verbal. But she never swears at me or kicks me again. We develop an unspoken respect for one another. Actually, it's quite remarkable.

Marlena lives in two places: her bed and her chair. Her entire day and all her nights are inside that one room. She has been in this room for five and a half years. She has not been in a wheelchair or out of the house for the last four of those years. The only way to transport her from her bed to her chair and back again is by using a Hoyer Lift. Sliding a large netting under her body and then stringing the netting with her body to a large wench-like machine, the Lift is continually cranked while her body is lifted higher and higher. After reaching the desired height, she is swung over to the next position and lowered. It is extremely frightening for the person being lifted, as they have absolutely no control over their movements. They are at the complete mercy of the person raising and lowering the Lift. For one such as Marlena who is helpless **and** blind, it must terrifying.

I'd been told to prepare myself for more kicking in the stomach from Marlena and for much screaming during this process.

I work very slowly with the Hoyer Lift. I also put one hand underneath Marlena's body so that she feels physically supported. In doing so, I try to create the sense that she is being held by my hands and not left to float helplessly and aimlessly in the air. I use my firm touch to convey that she is safe, that I will not hurt her … that she will not fall.

I speak ever so gently to her the entire time, letting her know exactly what I am doing each step along the way, "Marlena, I'm going to move you from this bed to your chair. Then you will be able to have a nice breakfast. I am going to work very slowly so that you do not feel afraid."

Keeping her usual refrain from conversation, she lets out a deep moan.

"I am sliding the blanket under you now. You don't need to do anything." In fact, I know she is unable to do anything. I merely want to assure her that I have control of the situation and she is completely safe.

"I am moving the blanket a little more. A little more now. Good. That's good. I am going to move it a little more. We are almost there. Thank you so much for your patience."

Moving to the opposite side of her body, "Marlena, now I am going to pull the blanket so it is completely under you. Just a little. Good. It's moving. Very good. One more pull and we'll have it.

Now, I am going to raise you up a little bit higher. Don't be afraid, Marlena. I am holding you underneath. Do you feel my hand underneath you? Good, Marlena. We are doing very well. You and I know how to do this. You are very safe with me. You are okay. I am taking good care of you.

Now, I am going to raise you a little bit higher. Just an inch or so. Do you feel my hand underneath you? Good, Marlena. We are doing very well. You and I know how to do this. You are very safe with me. You are okay. I am taking good care of you.

Don't be afraid, Marlena. I am holding you underneath. Do you feel my hand underneath you? Good, Marlena. We are doing very well. You and I know how to do this. You are very safe with me. You are okay. I am taking good care of you.

Now, I am going to raise you a little bit higher. Just an inch or so. Do you feel my hand underneath you? Good, Marlena. We are doing very well. You and I know how to do this. You are very safe with me. You are okay. I am taking good care of you.

Don't be afraid, Marlena. I am holding you underneath. Do you feel my hand underneath you? Good, Marlena. We are doing very well. You and I know how to do this. You are very safe with me. You are okay. I am taking good care of you.

Now, I am going to raise you a little bit higher. Just an inch or so. Do you feel my hand underneath you? Good,

Marlena. We are doing very well. You and I know how to do this. You are very safe with me. You are okay. I am taking good care of you.

Let's rest a minute. You are safe. You are totally supported. You are okay. I am going to move you towards the chair just a little bit. Very very slowly now. How are you? Are you okay? I'm holding you. You are supported. You are safe.

Let's rest a minute. You are safe. You are totally supported. You are okay. I am going to move you a little bit more towards the chair. Very very slowly now. How are you? Are you okay? I'm holding you. You are supported. You are safe.

Let's rest a minute. You are safe. You are totally supported. You are okay. I am going to move you a little bit more towards the chair. Very very slowly now. How are you? Are you okay? I'm holding you. You are supported. You are safe. Here is your chair, Marlena. I am going to lower you on your chair. It's okay. I will move very slowly.

I am lowering you into your chair right now. Just a little bit. You are safe. We are doing very well. You are okay. I am supporting you. Do you feel my hand underneath you? You are not going to fall. You are safe with me.

A little more now. I am lowering you a little more. You are safe. You are okay. Now, here is your chair. You are sitting in your chair right now. You are okay."

She doesn't scream. She isn't terrified. I feel as if this is a great accomplishment for myself and for her.

The simple process of moving Marlena from the bed to her chair takes us close to an hour. It could have been done in minutes. After all, it is merely a matter of inserting the netting under her body, raising her up and swinging her to her chair. But this slow approach offers her the gift of safety. My touch under her body offers the gift of security. And she doesn't scream. She isn't terrified. If taking this much time means alleviating some emotional suffering for her, it is definitely worth the effort.

And, anyway, what else do we have to do today?

Little Jenny Gilman

*I*DON'T KNOW WHAT TO EXPECT. THIS IS MY first formal interview with a client I'll call Little Jenny Gilman. Jenny is 4 feet 5 inches tall, 87 years old and weighs about 90 pounds wet. She defies her age by bouncing through the house like a rubber ball on espresso. The love of her life is Gaston, who follows her around like a puppy dog. Actually Gaston is a puppy dog: a mangy French Poodle with a schizophrenic disposition.

Jenny has Alzheimer's disease and has recently lost her husband. There is only one relative of Jenny's who is still alive. He is older than Jenny and wants no part of her care. He is interviewing for a full time caregiver.

Jenny's home can be described in three words: Drab. Worn. Dirty. Everything is either beige or brown and has been in the house for years. Beige carpet, rotted and torn. Beige sofa, ripped and sprayed on by Jenny's dog, Gaston. Kitchen counter tiled in small beige squares with grout turned black through years of neglect. A bedroom decorated with a dark beige quilt and a crusty comforter that hasn't seen a washing machine in a very long time.

The "interview" is more of a visit and an opportunity to see how Jenny and I interact with each other. Jenny is energetic and sweet. We like each other. I am hired for 24-hour care with her: this means staying day and night five days in a row in this drab and dirty home. Although not required, and without compensation, I will spend many hours in the upcoming weeks cleaning the environment so that it feels healthy for Jenny and me.

This is my first experience with someone who has Alzheimer's and I don't know what to expect.

This is my first experience with someone who has Alzheimer's and I don't know what to expect. Jenny's brother-in-law who hires me does not explain much, most likely because he has little knowledge himself of the situation. My care for Jenny will be my first of many "on the job trainings."

One of the most obvious of Jenny's qualities is her exuberant energy. She loves to walk. She has a quick snappy little bounce to her gait. She sports the stamina of an athlete and can out-walk most of my friends. During our many long treks together, people easily notice and remark about her darling happy face, laughing blue eyes and tender demeanor. She likes to shop and takes my hand, holding it like a small child. Passers-by glance at us and smile, thinking we are mother and daughter. Around town in the Strip Malls there is still an occasional phone booth and Jenny always stops to scrape for a few coins. It must be a long-practiced habit.

Little Jenny Gilman loves to help in the kitchen. Her favorite work is paring asparagus. She positions herself at the counter with a soft butter knife in her right hand and a crisp new asparagus in her left. Deftly she pares all the little nibs from a tender asparagus, giving this activity her full and complete attention. She even bounces at the kitchen counter. I love seeing her in action at the sink.

Jenny's cooking has apparently been monitored for a long time. Her Kenmore stove has been permanently altered and the only way to operate it is to know the whereabouts of the secret valve that controls the flow of gas to the oven and stovetop.

Other alterations have been made to her home: a chain link fence skirts the circumference of her charred lawn and a large Master lock keeps Jenny from escaping her home and roaming the streets by herself.

Her house is filthy. That first week I am with Jenny, I spend many hours cleaning the refrigerator. Meat and poultry are spoiled because they have been left unwrapped in the freezer section along with several bags of garbage. Vegetables and fruit grow mold in the temperature-controlled bins. Milk sours. Meat rots. This is a lesson for me: never accept food from an elderly person I don't know.

Jenny's little puppy-dog loves only her. Gaston is incredibly gentle with her and no one else can get near that dog. He follows Jenny closer than her own shadow. Gaston defecates anywhere he pleases. Jenny gets toilet

paper to clean the dog's anus and actually inserts her
fingers up the dog's rectum. When I first see this, I am
close to vomiting. This cannot be allowed. There are several discussions with Jenny's brother-in-law about how
to deal with Gaston. We try a few of them, hoping that
Jenny can change her ways, but, ultimately, we have to
find a new home for the dog. This just about kills Jenny.
Her happy little spirit becomes so depressed after her
puppy dog, Gaston, disappears.

For many days and many nights, she wanders through
the house, wailing, "Gaston! Gaston! Where are you, my
little Gaston?"

She is pitiful. I am incredibly sad for her. My heart
feels sickened by the whole experience. Keeping the dog
was a choice that was extremely unhealthy for Jenny.
Finding a new home for Gaston broke her heart. With
her disease, Jenny cannot ascertain the benefits of finding a good home for her puppy dog. It's a "no win—no
win" situation.

Is there anything at all I can do to comfort her?

After a couple trial and error situations, I find that
Jenny's grief can be assuaged by a gentle scalp massage.
As she sits in her chair, I gently work my fingers through
her wiry grey hair. I massage her head and rub her neck
muscles. She finds this extremely soothing and often falls
fast asleep under my touch.

Jenny has one seemingly unusual diversion. She absolutely delights in pretty clothes. All the closets in each
of her three bedrooms are stuffed with designer cloth-
ing that she collected and saved through the years. Jenny
loves nylon stockings and has over four large dresser

drawers filled with them. She will put on one pair, then layer another and then another, leaving the ends of them hanging from her toes. Then she adds another pair and twists them and curls them into knots, wrapping and twirling them around her lower legs and ankles. She revels in this knotting behavior. Because she seems to get so much joy from this, I see no reason to stop her. But after awhile, she'll get frustrated with herself. When this is no longer fun for her, we find something new to do.

I often take Little Jenny to visit my 72 year old mother who lives nearby. She is always happy on these outings and surprises me with an astonishing memory of where my mother lives. Alzheimer's is like that: at times, the person affected does not exhibit any signs of the disease at all.

I treat Jenny like my own child. I buy her a baby-doll that looks remarkably like a newborn infant. She is totally enthralled by this "baby." She loves this little doll. She nicknames her "Susie." Jenny holds her and strokes her round face and tenderly talks to her as if it were alive. She brings her to meals. She lays her by her side at bed-time. She talks to her and hugs her. I have the most precious photo of Jenny holding Susie on her lap and gazing at her. She has the sweet look of a new grandmother seeing her grandchild for the first time. Sweetly innocent. Delicious. Wondrously beautiful.

I care for Jenny for almost eleven months. During this time, the Alzheimer's disease steadily progresses. Jenny's behavior declines and changes in mean aggressive ways. Her happy demeanor can change instantly to volatile outbursts. I question myself. Has she grown tired of me? Am I doing something wrong in my care for her? Is there something I don't understand? Do I need to get more help?

I talk with professionals who are familiar with the disease. I read everything I can find on Alzheimer's. I learn about the changes in a person's behavior and I do not take it personally when Jenny's needs are beyond my capabilities. It's a sad day for me when I realize that I can no longer care for her. Eventually she is placed in a home designed for persons in advanced stages of Alzheimer's disease.

I will miss Little Jenny. I will miss our walks and her laughing eyes. I will miss our times together at the kitchen counter preparing meals. The day she is moved into an Institution, I pack a small bag for her. I fill it with lots of nylon stockings. I tuck Baby Susie under her arm and kiss her good-bye.

She reaches out her hand to me. She thinks we are going for a walk.

I quickly turn and slip away from her, not wanting her to see my tears.

A Post-It-Note Life

*T*HE POST-IT-NOTES ARE A DEAD GIVE-
away:

"This gift came from Victoria at Christmas in 2001" is taped behind the sculpture on the coffee table.

"Call Dr. Wickford every March to schedule cholesterol check" is taped to the calendar.

"This picture taken when we went to Mount Shasta in 1999."

"Ellen at the electric company was rude when I told her about my lights flicking on and off. Ask for someone else next time." March 3, 2004.

"Tell my neighbor, Susan, about weekend plans."

"Jimmy's picture when he was a teenager. It was taken in 1961. He looks like Johnny Cash." February 6, 2001

The refrigerator is a regular time organizational system:

Put out the trash on Tuesday.

Give the phone bill to Susie.

Take Fosamex every Tuesday—no food for an hour afterwards.

Don't lay down for 1 hour after taking Fosamex.

Dial-A-Ride comes on Thursday for a trip to the doctors for Iron infusion.

Of course, there are the required phone numbers:

Emergency 911

Gas Co (1) (800) 455-9977

Electric Co (1) (800) 322-6756

Telephone 449-2333

Susie (1) (909) 857-5878

Jimmy (1) (404) 665-3422

Neighbor—Jackie 449-2332

Dr. Lynn 449-8621

Dentist 449-3309

Some post-it-notes are dated as far back as 14 years ago.

The condo has a stunning location. Hanging over a Monterey cliff, it offers the sound of the surf as it crashes under the stiff pylons. There's a small patio garden speckled with California coastal favorites: pink impatiens, orchids not yet in bloom, popping purple fuchsias and the required ferns. Simple. Tasteful. Understated.

The diminutive figure that greets me doesn't resent my being there. Well, at least not in the beginning. He takes kindly to me as if I'm an old friend he's known for many many years.

His balding head, deep brown eyes and missing eyebrows give him the appearance of an aging tired owl. His wiry frame is chiseled and lean. At 5 feet 10 inches, he can't weigh more than 140 pounds. He moves quickly with his walker but his eyes are blank.

This client has been assigned to me through a conservator. Jerry had been out wandering the neighborhood and fell one night. He was admitted to a hospital where he spent three days hooked up to life support after internal hemorrhaging. He has no living relatives. No known friends. The conservator is just getting to know him, his condition and his needs. At this point, care is almost a crapshoot because there is little history available on the client. It is only later that possible psychosis, Alzheimer's and dementia will be considered. Wanting for a diagnosis, I'll refer to his condition as Alzheimer's.

I walk into this new situation and all I know is Jerry's age, height, weight and need for food and personal care.

"Would you like a cup of coffee?" he asks.

"That would be very nice," I respond.

It doesn't seem odd to him that, although this is the first time I've ever seen him, I search through his cupboards for coffee, filters and coffee cups. Preparing our morning java, I locate a couple of spoons, some sugar and coffee creamer. Poking around, I notice there is nothing sharp in any of the kitchen drawers. There is only one knife and it's a butter knife. No kitchen shears. No skewers for BBQ's. No carving knives.

Nothing sharp. Nothing pointed. Nothing that could puncture anyone. This is a room that says, "Watch my back."

So noted.

I begin to prepare our coffee. I've been working with the sick and dying long enough to quickly and seamlessly blend into my client's environment as if I've lived there for years. Without exception, in every single home where I've worked, everyone places kitchen utensils and food items in predictable places. In a matter of minutes, I've figure out that his morning meal consists of either eggs or oatmeal. I inquire as to which one he would like this fog-laced morning.

"Oh, you're my guest! Yet, you are fixing me breakfast. How very thoughtful of you. Yes, yes, the eggs will be fine."

> **Unexpectedly, as quickly as a child's spinning top jumps out of control, Jerry turns on me.**

Unexpectedly, as quickly as a child's spinning top jumps out of control, Jerry turns on me.

"GET MY COFFEE!" he hollers.

"Where's my coffee? Get my eggs!!! I'm hungry!!! Get my eggs now!!! Give me something to eat!!! Don't we have anything to eat? Where's my food!!! I need some water!!! Hurry!!! I'm hungry!!! I need some food now!!! Get my coffee!!!"

Sometimes medication makes clients voraciously hungry. Sometimes in an angry Alzheimer's client, hunger can be a trigger.

Jerry's agitation escalates quickly. As always, I go inward for guidance. Listening to the voice of my intuition, I very slowly approach Jerry with his coffee. As I begin to set the cup in front of him, I gently rest my free hand on his left shoulder. I feel him relax under my touch.

I continue to prepare his breakfast. As fast as I can hand him a cup, plates and bowls of food, that's as fast as he devours it. I am amazed at the amount of food this small thin frame can hold. A banana, a cinnamon roll and two slices of cheese keep him quiet while I fry two slices of bacon, scramble three eggs and toast two slices of bread. While gorging on the food, Jerry inhales a glass of orange juice and two cups of coffee.

Inside the orange juice, an assigned visiting nurse has hidden liquid doses of anti-psychotic medicine that have been prescribed to help temper his erratic behavior.

Once his hunger is satiated, Jerry piles plates, bowls, coffee cup one on top of the other creating a ceramic mountain that makes me a bit nervous. He's jittery. I stay very close pretending not to. With his long thin fingers he raises the mountain of dishes to the cracked turquoise tiled counter and clink clink they splat on the tile. They don't break. I mentally say a prayer of gratitude for this bit of good fortune. I count my blessings. As inconsequential as it may seem, this may be as good as it gets today.

He pushes himself away from the low counter that serves as his dining table. Grabbing his best support, the walker, he lugs his heavy swollen feet and shuffles off through the living room, past the musty hall and into the bathroom where he begins to stare at himself in the pitted freckled mirror.

I follow Jerry into the bathroom. I put on fresh gloves. It's time for his morning shower. He's resistant.

One learns quickly that reasoning and reminding are not useful communication tools when dealing with someone who appears to have Alzheimer's or dementia. Often, it helps to gently proceed with the task at hand while engaging in pleasant light conversation. So, instead of talking about giving Jerry a shower, I simply continue as if he has already agreed to have one.

I turn on the water.

"Is the water warm enough, Jerry? Would you like it a little cooler?"

My line of reckoning does not work.

"No. I don't need a shower. I just took one."

We do manage some oral hygiene. Again, I gently rest my hand on his shoulder. Jerry takes a deep breath. I rub his tight muscles under my left hand as I coax the old spotted dentures from his drawn face using my right hand. There's a dish near the bathroom sink. Its only purpose is to soak Jerry's teeth. There's a little pop pop fizz fizz as I place his fragile dentures into the plastic receptacle bubbling with the magic denture disk. It hisses. I remove my gloves and apply fresh ones. There's a once-white washcloth as old as Jerry's dentures on a thin stainless steel towel bar. He grabs at it before I've had time to warm the water and wet the cloth.

All of a sudden, like a spring uncoiling, Jerry lunges toward the commode. Those huge swollen feet seem lithe and light. It's time for the ever-coveted bowel movement. His face relaxes as he relieves himself. He's suddenly very still and very quiet.

He's confused. He doesn't know what to do next. He's unable to clean himself. I warm some handy-wipes to get the job done with some ease and comfort. More fresh gloves. Jerry wears a catheter full time. The nurse has requested special cleaning and care of his penis. He's uncircumcised, so I need to pull back the foreskin and apply an anti-fungal cream so bacteria doesn't back up into the bladder and cause an infection. More on the job training.

I've learned to use every opportunity as it arises: he's at the toilet, pants off and it's a good time for peri-care. Fresh gloves to apply adult diaper. I add undershorts over the "Depends" and this is another golden flash of inspiration. This makes Jerry feel very grown up and every bit of self-confidence is a blessing for him.

More fresh gloves. Wash Jerry's hands again. Insert the now-clean dentures. There is that morning ooze seeping from his right eye. Clean the debris and apply a bit of RX cream. Comb what little hair he has.

He's quite done with me now. He's taken all he can.

With strong lungs, he yells at me, "Let me go! Leave me alone. I have to lay down. Don't bother me. Where's my robe? I want to go to bed. Leave me alone. What are you doing? Why are you here? Leave me alone."

Another bumbling shuffle through the hall and he waddles to his room. He lays down.

Good. He's resting. Maybe now I can have my morning coffee. Before you can say, "Folgers French Roast," he's up again, grumbling and shuffling and heading for the kitchen, yelling, "Where's my coffee? Get my eggs!!! I'm hungry!!! Get my eggs now!!! Give me something to eat!!! Don't we have anything to eat? Where's my food!!! I need some water!!! Hurry!!! I'm hungry!!!"

In an advanced Alzheimer's client who shows signs of combative, psychotic behavior, the key rule is, "Avoid confrontation." Since Jerry already ate breakfast but is hollering for another, I go along with his request. Again, I bring out orange juice, make oatmeal, fry an egg and some bacon. He happily devours his second breakfast of the day.

This is how Jerry spends his day: Shuffle. Shuffle. Eat. Shuffle. Shuffle. Go to the bathroom. Shuffle. Shuffle. Shuffle. Lay down. Shuffle. Shuffle. Shuffle. Eat. Shuffle. Shuffle. Shuffle. Eat. Go to the bathroom. Shuffle. Shuffle. Shuffle.

Television doesn't interest him. Neither does music, taking a walk outside, sitting on the patio, flipping through a magazine or playing cards. The phone rings. He answers it. He can't understand what is going on. This frustrates him. His day is boring. Jerry is angry.

Our day wears on. At 4:00 PM a social worker visits. Preliminary investigation into Jerry's past has been made. A few of his neighbors have been contacted. The social worker offers her wisdom. She advises that Jerry used to have many friends. Keeping him social is important. He will be much happier and more content if he maintains social interaction.

"What do you suggest?" I ask.

"I've brought some coloring books and crayons. Maybe you could color with him."

"Right. Why don't you color with him and I'll run around telling other caregivers to color with their clients so they'll remain social." This I do not say.

"Settle down, Jean." I say to myself. "You just need your morning coffee."

"I certainly will do my best, Mrs. Johnson."

Not only have I not had my morning coffee, I will not have coffee this day. I will be lucky to have time to eat a meal. Nor will I sleep in three nights.

Jerry's routine at night is, in fact, more difficult than his days. It appears that he has a condition called "Sundowners"—a form of Alzheimer's in which a person becomes very agitated, confused and angry once the sun goes down. Often they are terrified of the dark and will stay up all night long out of fear of falling asleep.

This was definitely Jerry's situation. Once the sun went down, he would slink and shuffle between his room and mine. He quietly entered my room as I attempted to sleep. He would appear at my bedside without warning. I'd wake up, often gasping, to find him lording over me, glaring at me and yelling, "Wake up! Wake up!"

"Jerry, it's time to sleep. It's bedtime. Go back to bed and rest."

He would. For 10 minutes. Some times 15 minutes on a long stretch. By the second night, I am drained to the point of feeling like I've caught some mental condition myself. Jerry's ghostlike presence, his creeping through the house in the dark, his hanging over my bedside, his hollering at me saps me of the little strength I have left after the 15 hour day of caring for him. At the start of a new day, when I am supposed to be fresh and alert, keeping him safe from harm, and watching for any sign of danger from him, thus protecting myself, I am pie-eyed and exhausted.

On the third day, and, long overdue, I decide I need to admit I have worked beyond my physical limits and make a call for a replacement caregiver. The conservator is understanding and will find someone to relieve me as soon as she can. Only moments later, as I change his diaper, Jerry gouges deeply into my forearms with his strong thick nails.

I guess this is Jerry's way of telling me how much he'll miss me.

Death by Dying

*T*HEY WEAR THEIR 50 YEARS TOGETHER like loose robes. They glide through each others lives with the ease and comfort of friends that have known each other since childhood. They are both short of stature, yet his five foot five inches towers over her little five-foot frame. Even in her eighties, she could be a ballerina. At least, that's what Lewis says. He loves her so much. This is so obvious, you can't miss it. The way he says her name: like it is the name of a young princess he has the privilege to serve. The way he tilts his head to hear what she says. The way he holds her hand as if he's been just handed a newborn kitten that he adores.

She is the quietest person I have ever met. Her diminutive voice is more like a warm whisper. It briefly crosses my mind that she is so soft spoken because she is dying and feels very weak. But Lewis tells me that Mary has always spoken this way. She was always this gentle. Always sweet. Always non-demanding.

Mary lies in bed so very still. The entire six days I am here, I rarely hear a peep out of her. She asks for nothing.

She has a tiny little smile that matches her tiny little voice. She is incredibly soft. If I have to pick one word to describe her, it would be "feather." So soft. So gentle. Like the down feather of a baby bird. I think a strong wind could scoop her up and whisk her away.

I nickname her "Trouble-Maker." For obvious reasons.

I nickname her, "Trouble-Maker." For obvious reasons.

Mary likes her nickname. When I need to change her or spoon feed her or turn her body so that bed sores do not develop, she will very slowly turn her head towards me and say with the softest of sounds, "Am I being a Trouble-Maker?" This always puts a smile on my face. And she likes knowing that she's made me smile.

Lewis and Mary live in understated luxury. Lewis had made his fortune years ago in the movie industry. There was plenty of help to keep their fine home in tip top shape: a pool service, several gardeners and a house-keeper. He was a production manager and had worked on some major films. His fame does not seem to affect his ego and he is gracious, kind and attentive. Mary has been set up in a separate bedroom for her final days and Lewis is constantly stepping inside to see how she is doing.

They do not have any children and I never found out if this was by choice or fate.

Lewis and Mary's story here is not a big drama. It is the calm account of two people who spent many years together. Without knowing their past, I witnessed an immense love between the two of them. A love that manifested itself in little tender glances. In kind words. In a grasp of fingertips.

When I am with the dying—be it for a day or several months— I become acutely aware of every single breath a person takes. When Mary died, her last breath was so silent and so gentle that it was almost imperceptible. She took a breath. She did not take another. She died that easily. That simply. That willingly. That beautifully. She was laying in bed on her back. Her eyelids were shut. Her breathing very soft. I thought she was dozing off to sleep.

If people die as they live, Mary must have had a lovely life. She must have been a soul rich in peace and deep contentment.

Lewis was not in the room. Mary passed so quickly that I did not have time to call him until it was too late. I went to find him and told him that Mary was gone.

This wonderful kind loving man began to wail with an angst and grief that pulled at my heartstrings in a way that I ached all over. He moved to Mary's bedside letting his tears pour over her little frame. He held her frail lifeless little body, begging her to come back, begging her not to go, begging her to stay. Begging and sobbing. Sobbing and hoping she'd smile up at him. Sobbing and hoping she'd whisper "Hello, Lewis." Sobbing and hoping Mary would whisper "I love you" just one more time.

&

Helping Others;
Helping Yourself

Loving
the Elderly and the Dying

*T*HERE IS MUCH THAT I HAVE LEARNED IN helping the aging and the dying. As life slowed for them—and, ultimately for me—so did my thinking. As my thinking slowed down, my intuition "spoke" louder and louder. This voice often gave me answers that otherwise eluded me through hours of research. I learned that I could truly trust my inner voice. I learned that wisdom—often called "insight" or "intuition"—was as available as my mind was quiet.

Working with the elderly or those who are dying draws on a different set of skills than our daily lives demand. We can feel unprepared and overwhelmed by the changes that occur as a loved one ages or begins to die. Know that you do not have to walk this journey alone. There are support groups for caregivers. Hospice organizations are an invaluable source of information, guidance and support for the dying. There are even massage classes that can teach you various techniques for working with the elderly and the dying.

In the following pages, I have shared some general ideas with you that I hope you will find helpful. Drawing on my experience from massage therapy through the years, I adapted certain "ways of being" with my massage clients and translated them into my care of the elderly and the dying. I have also included some very simple massage techniques that you might find beneficial.

Walk Softly ... Talk Softly

*W*HEN SOMEONE IS VERY ILL OR DYING, his or her entire body is undergoing a metamorphosis. The systems in the body begin to slow down. Bodily functions change. Sometimes they shut down completely. Noises seem louder. Scents are more pronounced. Many elderly can no longer see very well and their hearing may be compromised. The mind may not be able to process huge amounts of information.

Have you ever had a cold or had the flu and had a well-meaning friend barge into your home or bellow into your ear? The friend intends to convey good wishes. Instead, you feel like you've been emotionally assaulted.

It is not necessary to overcompensate for someone's loss of hearing or seeing unless the person who is ill requests that you do so. Your demeanor says as much about your care for them as your words do.

Intention is a powerful tool ...

I believe that it is best to approach the elderly and the dying with an awareness that their bodies are changing.

Walk with purpose but step softly. Let them know by the way you approach them that you are here to offer any comfort you can.

Intention is a very powerful tool. Before entering any room, I mentally think positive thoughts about what I hope to communicate. Some people call this praying. Something as simple as, "May my presence bring peace and comfort to my loved one" can set a tone for the entire time you spend together.

The Wonderful World of Touch

*F*OR THE ELDERLY AND THE DYING, TOUCH can be a way of communicating that transcends words. Dying persons process life at a very rapid rate as they approach their final days. They experience anxiety, guilt, and fear. They worry about their loved ones, their finances, and the act of dying itself. Various drugs can exacerbate their feelings of depression and hopelessness.

Compassionate touch communicates that you care … that the elderly or dying person is not alone … that "we are in this together." Touch can soften a harsh moment and ease an uncomfortable situation. When words fail, touch speaks volumes.

Touch is a simple yet powerful gift. Touch gives to the giver as it gives to the receiver! It makes us feel good that we can do something very nice for the person who is ill or dying.

You can usually find a way to safely and meaningfully touch everyone: it may be by touching the person's scalp, hands or feet. Rarely do I meet someone who does not like to be touched at all. As a caregiver, I always ask permission before I touch someone I do not know very well.

Many people tire of being by the bedside of their ill and dying friends and family. They feel useless. They feel helpless to do anything worthwhile. They may have "talked themselves out." But touch usually *always* feels good. Rarely does someone tire of this type of comfort. And caregivers feel deep satisfaction in knowing that they are truly offering something valuable to their loved one. It gives the patient a time of relaxation and a feeling of being deeply connected to the one who is providing the "massage." It's win-win for everyone.

Touch can communicate far more than words. Know, however, that there may be instances when touch is not advisable. Some of these may include the following:

- Certain medications cause the skin to become very thin and to tear easily
- Bruises or cuts
- Certain heart conditions
- Sore joints, arthritis
- Open wounds
- Thrombosis

I always get a doctor's approval before providing massage to a client. I advise you to do the same.

The way that you touch begins with your first contact with a person. How you walk into the room sets the tone. If you are harried or irritated, the elderly and the dying will know. Their instincts are open and fresh like a child's and they will sense that your mood is "off." Step softly, yet firmly.

Your tone of voice conveys your state of mind. Too loud a voice can be overwhelming to those who are suffering. Too soft a voice may not be heard. Modulate your voice in a gentle calm manner. Speak slowly, especially for those who may be hard of hearing or hard of understanding.

Touch can communicate that we are in this together.

The actual moment of touch is very important. Whether or not you are aware, your energy accesses the energy body of another long before you make actual physical contact with them. Approach the person you are going to touch in a slow steady manner. Gently place your hand on the area that you are going to hold, stroke or massage. Now, you are ready to begin. On the next two pages, I offer a couple of ways in which you can provide love, support and comfort through the magical gift of your touch.

Scalp Massage

*A*AAAAAAH . . . . . ." "Mmmmmmm . . . . ."
Oooooh . . . ." These are some of the lovely sounds
you'll hear when providing a scalp massage. I believe that
a scalp massage is so effective because it is being applied
to one of the *busiest* parts of our bodies: that protective
container for our never-quiet brain! Massaging the scalp
truly can help the elderly and the dying to let go of all
their wearisome thoughts and help them relax.

Scalp massage is a wonderful way to provide touch to
another. No one needs to undress for this type of massage. Scalp massage feels very safe for most people. The
scalp is easily accessible: all one needs to do is to stand or
sit at the side of the person receiving the scalp massage.
If the person is bed ridden, a scalp massage can easily be
given from the back of the bed and won't interfere with
oxygen tubes and other equipment that might be connected to the patient. Rarely is there any reason not to
touch the scalp, unless, of course, in cases of head injuries.

Scalp massage is easy to apply. Simply imagine you
are washing the person's hair. Play with a variety of

techniques: long slow finger strokes, short quicker strokes, strokes applied with or without some pressure. If the person has enough hair, glide some of the strands through your fingertips.

Scalp massage feels very safe for most people.

Even a gentle tug at the hair can feel good, but go lightly with this technique.

Let your fingers do the walking! Move your hands over your loved one's scalp with tenderness and devotion. Be firm in your touch, but not rough. Visualize strength coming through your fingertips, but do not force pressure. You may even experiment with closing your eyes during this process. Feeling without seeing will add a new dimension to your touch. Try it and notice the results. Let the relaxation and sounds from your loved one provide you with information as to how much value you are providing. Enjoy giving this type of massage and your loved one will feel the satisfaction and comfort through every pore.

Face Massage

*I*LOVE STROKING THE FACE. IT FEELS LIKE such a loving gesture. Face massage is easy and uncomplicated. You might begin by making small circles with your fingertips over the cheeks and the chin. Make circles across the forehead. Give the forehead extra attention. So many people scrunch their faces and hold worry and tension in their foreheads. Simple gestures like long wide strokes across the forehead with your fingers can be delicious! I also like to draw lines from the bridge of the nose up to the top of the forehead. I actually count to myself as I do this and attempt to be patient enough to "draw" 21 lines. If someone is having trouble falling asleep, this tender technique can be a wonderful way to help him relax.

Do not underestimate these simple, genuine forms of solace.

You might even add some words to your massage. Here are a few sample choices that would be appropriate:

"Just close your eyes and relax."

"No worries. Just relax and let go of all your thoughts."

"There's nothing for you to do. Nothing to say. You can rest now."

Finally, know that even very gentle forms of touch can communicate a sense of safety, caring and connection. There may be a time when massage is not appropriate. Simply holding hands with a loved one can send a powerful message of comfort. Do not underestimate these simple genuine forms of solace.

When All Else Fails

$\mathcal{B}$EING WITH A LOVED ONE WHO IS DYING can put a strain on our heartstrings. Even if the relationship with one who is terminally ill is a good one, we are processing so many feelings at one time that we can feel overwhelmed.

But when the relationship with one who is dying is ragged, tattered or fraught with past guilt, trauma or abuse, being with the dying person can be especially difficult.

In some instances, we want to be close and affectionate with the dying person and our behavior is not welcome.

We may want to clear the air on old situations that need completion, but a person may have had a stroke or been in a serious accident and can no longer verbally communicate.

Intention is at the heart of communication. In those instances where you cannot share openly with someone or physical touch is not welcome or existent in the relationship, I believe that one can share "heart to heart". By this, I mean to say, that you can speak in your silence to the heart and soul of the one who is ill or dying. You can share your wishes for comfort. You can share your wishes for peace of mind. You can share your love. I believe that at some level the ill and the dying will receive your messages. So do not hold back your heart from them. Speak out loud if you can. Say what you need to say and share your feelings when you can. When you cannot share aloud, whisper from your heart and soul. The spirit of your loved one will receive your kindness and your care. Know that you are heard and be at peace knowing that you have done and said all that you can.

Caregivers Have Needs, Too

*Y*OUR FRIENDS HAVE TOLD YOU, YOUR doctor has told you, and your neighbor has told you. Now, I am going to tell you: take care of yourself. You can't give from an empty cup. Refuel so you have something to give.

When you are a caregiver, you are expending a huge amount of emotional energy, physical attention, and spiritual stamina. As the person you are caring for continues to decline, more and more of your reserves are being used. You may feel overwhelmed with the challenges before you. You may be thrown into situations for which you have no tools. You may feel helpless or at the very least, ineffective. Often, this happens so imperceptibly, that one reaches full-blown burnout before saying, "I think I need a time out."

I have been with loved ones who stay up night after night with their dying relatives, terrified that they will not be with them for their final moments. I have seen families stay for days on end with a dying loved one, only to leave the home and have their loved one pass away a few hours later. They feel guilty that they have somehow failed.

Refuel so you have something to give.

I offer a few suggestions on the following pages that I hope will benefit you. Please read them with an open mind and a full heart.

Live Guilt Free

MANY YEARS AGO AS I WAS WORKING through my new role as a single parent, plagued with guilt that I was not doing a good job, my therapist taught me something. She said that guilt is not actually a human emotion, like fear, joy, anger and delight. Guilt is actually not a feeling at all. It is a totally *manufactured* experience and is the result of something we have been taught. This information helped me immensely. Whenever, I feel guilty, I know this is not a true feeling. I can dismiss those "guilty thoughts" as old information—usually passed on to me by one who wanted something from me that I could not give them.

Now, when I know I need to take care of myself, I see this knowledge as a gift for those whose care is in my hands. When I refuel, I have so much more to happily give them.

Sleep

*L*ACK OF SLEEP IS ONE OF THE MOST COM-
mon areas where caregivers suffer. Avoid tempta-
tion to go through your days with less and less rest. Our
bodies and our minds actually recharge during sleep.
When I don't get enough rest, I become edgy, irritated
and impatient. I'm very clear now that without a good
night's rest, nothing works well for me.

If you are a caregiver hired through an Agency, keep
your communications clear with your supervisor especially when your work situation does not permit a full
night's sleep. You are their eyes and ears: let them know
what is going on. They will find a way to provide for
your needs.

If you are caring
for a loved one, plenty
of rest is essential for
you to function, to
make good decisions

**Plenty of rest is essential
for you to function well
during these trying times.**

and to be emotionally available. This does not mean
dozing off in a chair beside the bed of your loved one.

This means leaving the room, going to a quiet place and sleeping in a comfortable bed.

Know Your Boundaries

ONLY *YOU* KNOW WHEN TOO MUCH IS TOO much. Only *YOU* know how your body feels, if your mind is at rest and if your soul is peaceful. No one else can get inside of you to determine your needs or your limits. Be aware of when to "draw your line." Then, honor your limits.

Say "Yes" to those who want to help you. Delegate some of the responsibilities when help is offered. Ask for help. Let others have the joy of giving to you during this trying time.

Give to Your Body

*H*EALTHY FOODS PROVIDE ENERGY FOR the days ahead. Foods high in sugar will deplete you and possibly leave you feeling anxious. Avoid them. Drink lots of water.

Find ways to be pampered. I love massage. When my work schedule is heavy, I have no problem receiving a massage every week. I give with my hands ... it is a gift to be "given to" by well-trained and loving hands. You might benefit from a pedicure or a facial.

Do you like to dance? Play a sport? Go to the gym? Do you enjoy swimming? Taking a walk? Even a 20-minute walk outdoors can renew your spirit and give you a new perspective. Moving the body activates endorphins—those wonderful hormones that make us feel good.

Fill Your Soul

$\mathcal{B}$EING IN NATURE IS ONE OF THE BEST ways I know to bring peace to the soul. Again, a 20-minute walk may be just what your soul needs to relax and regain equanimity.

Meditation is another powerful gift to give yourself. There are many forms of meditation. I encourage you to try a couple and see what feels right for you.

Here is one of the simplest and one of my favorite forms:

Sit in a cross-legged position. If this is uncomfortable for you, sit on a chair with a good back support, feet flat on the floor, legs uncrossed.

- ⁓ Close your eyes.

- ⁓ Focus on your breath as you exhale: follow your breath as it leaves your nostrils and rests just above your upper lip.

- ⁓ With each breath you inhale, follow it with as much awareness as possible.

- ⁓ Continue to follow your breath each time you inhale and exhale.

This is a simple yet powerful way in which to totally relax your entire body.

Perhaps you have an inspirational book from which you can draw strength. Take a few minutes to open that book and soak up the strength it has to give you.

Be with people who support you.

Be with people who support you and with whom you can process your feelings.

Many people find keeping a journal a satisfying way to release their emotions. Don't be afraid to get professional help if you need it. Many American daily lives are not set up to easily access strong emotional supporters when needed. There are many support groups and professionals who can be a tremendous help to you right now. Use them gladly!

That Wonderful Elixer:
Gratitude

WORKING WITH THE ELDERLY AND THE dying teaches me a new sense of gratitude. Each day I am grateful for the gift of another day and the magic it brings. I am grateful for many things:

- the aroma of coffee brewing
- that wispy willowy cloud in the sky
- the scent of pine tress as I walk
- my son, Chris
- colors
- cranes
- chocolate
- my hairdresser
- my friend, Lois
- leaves
- lilies
- lavender
- pansies

~ poodles

~ pancakes

I actually spend some time towards the end of the day by writing in a journal in which I log at least one new "gratitude experience." It may be something I have seen or heard. A phone call from a friend. The way the sky looked at sunset today. Someone I met. A new insight. An emotional release. A change in attitude.

The act of writing anchors the gratitude in my psyche. It focuses my mind on those aspects of my life that are working. Writing out those experiences for which I am thankful is like watering the flowers instead of watering the weeds. I highly recommend it.

My Thanks to You

I WISH TO EXPRESS MY GRATITUDE TO YOU, My Readers.

Thank you for taking the time to read the words contained herein.

Thank you for your support of my efforts.

May the stories assist you in ways that are meaningful.

May you find suggestions that are helpful and practical.

May you glean a new understanding or a reinforcement of past knowledge that will enhance and add value to your life.

Please Share
Your Experiences with Others

*D*O YOU HAVE A PERSONAL STORY TO share? Are you now a professional caregiver or have you been cast in the role of caregiving for an ailing relative?

Have you had an experience with an aging friend or family member that you are willing to share with others?

Have you learned something about the dying process that might help someone else?

We are all in this together and we can learn from one another. Please reach out to others with your questions, your solutions and your personal stories through our blog at: www.CaregiversNook.com

Contact Information

Our virtual village
for care, comfort and compassion
for the elderly, the dying and their caregivers:

www.CaregiversNook.com
(website and blog)

Questions or Comments?

Are you ready to book a workshop?
Are you interested in becoming
a Resource available through our website?
Are you interested in bulk mail for shipping large orders?
Contact: jeannie@caregiversnook.com

For information about
A Caregiver's Winding Road
Seminars ◊ Book signings ◊ Workshops
Please email: jeannie@caregiversnook.com

A Caregiver's Winding Road
is available for purchase at:

www.CaregiversNook.com

online booksellers

and by order at your favorite bookstore

Thomas Enterprises
530c Alameda Del Prado, #194
Novato, California 94949

CPSIA information can be obtained at www.ICGtesting.com
Printed in the USA
LVOW042113100512

281155LV00001B/2/P